I0560388

For more information about our company, services, education programs, coach training, and consulting, please visit our website at

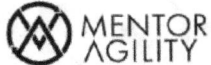

www.MentorAgility.com

Copyright 2024 Mentor Agility

Jackson Hole, Wyoming

All Rights Reserved

Mentor Agility © 2024

V1.2

ISBN:979-8-9853539-8-3

Printed in USA

Table of Contents

4

This page left blank

This page left blank

CHAPTER 1

READY, SET, GO!

The legend of Butch Cassidy, rooted in historical events, offers a rare glimpse into the past but also into ourselves. The end of an era known as the wild west, his story gives a glimpse into the origins of customs, traditions, and landmarks that shaped the western values of today.

Legends play a role in shaping and reinforcing a community's sense of identity. They provide a shared narrative that bind individuals together to create a sense of belonging within a culture. The legend of Butch Cassidy is no different. In the story of Butch Cassidy, we see the emergence of western values of self-reliance and community come together. Seemingly in conflict with each other, we come to learn that each value has its place in surviving a harsh landscape.

Legends have a remarkable ability to adapt and evolve over time, with variations of the story emerging as they are retold by different storytellers. This adaptability ensures that legends remain relevant and continue to resonate with audiences across different generations and cultural contexts. They serve as a rich tapestry of human imagination, history, and values, woven together to create an enduring narrative that becomes a mirror for us to see ourselves.

A measure of where we are in life, and where we are going, legends appeal to us because we can see ourselves within their woven tapestries. We will unravel the early days of Butch Cassidy in a series of short stories followed by journaling with guiding questions. These guiding questions will stimulate your critical reasoning and reflect upon how it relates to your journey of transformation. As you immerse yourself in the legend of Butch Cassidy, consider how it resonates with your own life experiences and the insights they offer.

We encourage you to open yourself up to the possibility of transformative change in your thinking, emotions, and decision-making. Remember, there are no right or wrong answers. Let your thoughts lead you to deeper insights.

Feel free to tap into your creativity through artistic expression. This isn't about creating masterpieces but rather it is a form of extended thinking. Whether through visual art or journal writing, this process unearths profound thoughts that propel us forward on our paths.

Writing down your insights acknowledges it to your soul, a very important step in healing emotional barriers and releasing thinking blocks outside your awareness while manifesting your goals. Through listening to yourself, without judging, changes a part of ourselves. Embrace the insights you gain, as they can pave the way for new perspectives and actions aligned with the life you envision.

To kick things off, set a personal or professional challenge to focus your experience through this journal. This challenge should be aligned with a goal or value you hold dear. Before jumping into the story of Butch Cassidy, take a moment to complete the three-step process outlined in the next chapter.

Thank you!

Ryan Elledge and Julie Elledge

CHAPTER 2

TRUE NORTH

The Swazi people have a rich cultural heritage where tracking is a vital skill for hunters and gathers. The term siswati refers to the entire process of following the footprints of an animal to find one's way back home. While it doesn't have a direct translation in English, it conveys the concept of navigating through the wilderness by reading and interpreting animal tracks to guide oneself to the goal and then back to familiar territory.

In this journal, A Journal Experience with Butch Cassidy, we will explore the wild landscape of the legend of Butch Cassidy, reading and interpreting our own tracks that will guide us back to the familiar territory of our own purpose and motivations. Along the way, guiding questions will provide the footprints that your soul that we do not always see unless we look for them.

The first step on your journey is to establish the challenge, or true north. The challenge, a three part process, serves as your true north. True north is crucial for accurately orienting maps, determining bearings, and navigating over long distances. When we undertake a journey of transformation, your personal inner compass, or guiding principles in life, symbolize your core values and aspirations that guide your decision making and actions. Whenever you feel lost, find your true north. It can be easy to get distracted in day-to-day living or in old habits, like explorers get lost in the woods. True north, your north star, comes out at night, in the darkness when it is the easiest to find your guide.

True North 3 Part Process

The three part process of establishing your true north is as follows:

The first step is to establish a Challenge. The challenge refers to a situation that requires effort, skill, or determination to overcome. They are an opportunity for growth, learning and development. The obstacles and difficulties you encounter while facing this challenge are the opportunities to demonstrate reliance and creativity to finding solutions.

The second step is to identify the Essential Question. The essential question gets to the root of underlying problem you need to solve. Underlying the challenge is a problem that needs to be solved. There will be many guiding questions to explore along your quest, because questions stimulate your critical reasoning. While problems can be seen as negative, they also represent opportunity to be creative. When developing your essential question you want to try and capture the over arcing driving question that needs to be answered for your challenge.

The third step is to formulate a Big Idea. Our values run silently in the background directing our decisions. By rooting your reflection in a big idea, it activates your motivation to act. To hope you with this process, we have identified four untranslatable words. An untranslatable word does not have a single word equivalent in English; however, it does have a far more descriptive explanation from another culture that we admire. Use the four untranslatable words as a jump off point to express the big idea or values behind your true north. Feel free to change or combine the words to fully express yourself, or abandon it completely and write your own big idea. There are no right or wrong ways to express yourself.

If you are like most people, you can list off a bunch of values, or choose them from a list easily enough. To dig a bit deeper, we need a story to really express what is the motivation behind your true north.

Let's get started.

1. Challenge:

Rewrite the following sentence as a challenge you would like to explore orr write your own if you would like. Be specific when you write your challenge and how it relates to a long-term goal.

Convert moments of self-doubt or hesitation into opportunities for self-reflection and growth, strengthening my resolve to pursue my goals.

2. Essential Question:

Questions wake up your critical reasoning. Modify the essential question, or change it completely, to fit with your challenge.

What is influencing me and how do I turn it into fuel for reaching my goals?

3. Big Idea: Circle one idea to guide your journaling.

Review the list of untranslatable words from another culture, considering their meanings and significance. Select one that resonates with your goal and essential question, or modify it to better suit your needs. If you prefer, write your own big idea.

1. *Fingerspitzengefühl* is a German term that translates to "fingertip feeling" or "intuitive flair" in English. It refers to the ability to handle situations with sensitivity, intuition, and tact, often in complex or delicate circumstances. This term is commonly used to describe someone who has a keen instinct or intuitive understanding of a situation, enabling them to make appropriate decisions or judgments. It implies a deep understanding that goes beyond mere knowledge or expertise, often involving an intuitive grasp of subtle nuances or intricacies.

2. *Sabsung* is a Thai term that refers to the feeling of being revitalized or rejuvenated by something that brings excitement, joy, or liveliness to one's life. It encapsulates the notion of finding inspiration, energy, or a sense of renewal through engaging in activities, experiences, or relationships that uplift and invigorate the spirit. It implies a positive transformation or a rekindling of enthusiasm for life.

3. *Kombinować* is a Polish term roughly translated as "to figure something out" or "to come up with a solution by thinking creatively or resourcefully." It implies using one's ingenuity, resourcefulness, or cleverness to devise a plan or solve a problem, often in a flexible or improvisational manner. (It can also carry connotations of scheming or devising a plan, sometimes in a slightly dubious or unconventional way.) Overall, *kombinować* reflects a proactive and adaptable approach to problem-solving or navigating tricky situations.

4. **Agon**, an ancient greek term, carries a rich and nuanced meaning. The word captures the dynamic tension between opposing forces and the inherent struggle individuals face in their pursuit of goals, ideals, or self-realization. Signify a broader struggle or conflict, it could be physical, intellectual, emotional, or spiritual. *Agon* emphasizes the complexity and intensity of human endeavor, highlighting both the adversities to overcome and the potential for growth and triumph through struggle and conflict.

Guiding Questions:

- What is your big idea?

- What does your true north mean to you?

- What do you believe you need to address to honor your true north?

CHAPTER 3

REPUTATION

The wind blew softly over the wide open plains. Spring gently coaxed the new growth out while the snow quietly retreated. It was a bright spring day like any other. Perhaps some people felt the ground shift, but most likely, no one took notice. It would be a couple of decades, maybe more, before people knew the significant of the boy born on April 13,1866. But it was the beginning of a life that would change the face of bank robbing.

Some people have since called him another Robin Hood. He was a friendly character who was rarely too busy to stop and give you his full attention. It's rumored he was well liked, known for always keeping his word and looked out for his neighbors. When folks less fortunate needed something, he was quick to give away what he had. What he earned honestly or what was stolen was of little matter to him or those he helped. Wild West magazine wrote about him. They said, "One boy, 10-year-old Vic Button, whose father managed the CS Ranch east of town where the outlaws camped, remembered Butch as a likable man with a broad grin. He said the outlaw gave him candy. Button also said that one day when he told Butch how much he admired his horse, Butch replied that someday he might give it to him. A few days later, Butch kept his word. Following the robbery, as the three outlaws were changing to fresh horses, Butch told the cowboy who had been attending the animals to give his winded horse to the young boy at the CS Ranch." When the law came looking for him, you bet they covered for him. If you haven't figured it yet, we're telling the legend of Butch Cassidy.

Guiding Questions:

- Take a moment and reflect on what stood out to you so far in this story.

- Butch Cassidy cared about those around him and helped them where he could. How do you help those around you?

- There is a lot of talk about Butch Cassidy over the last 160 some years. Some of its true and some of its not. He was a bank robber, leader of the Wild Bunch Gang, a mighty fine neighbor, and an outlaw. What do you hope people will say about you when you're gone?

- Why does it matter what folks say about you?

- How does your reputation relate to your true north discussed in Chapter 2?

CHAPTER 4
FINANCIAL WELL-BEING

Robert Leroy Parker was born to Anne Gillies and Maximillian Parker. Leroy, as Butch was known back then, was a likable kid. Bright and creative, little was beyond his inquisitive mind. In the evenings the joyous sounds of the harmonica could be heard from their little house as he entertained his host of siblings. As the oldest of 13 children, he was quick to finish his chores and help with the responsibility of taking care of his siblings.

Life out west was a glorious, untamed and brutal environment. There are many tales of the romantic cowboy riding off into the sunset but life could be harsh and short for those who were not smart and imaginative. Life came at you quick and stretched resources to the limit. Maximillian, father to the infamous boy, would take work far from home often being gone for long months leaving Leroy to help his mother at home. Leroy's family was poor and as such, he often found himself as the hired help for the ranches close to home. Young though he was, Leroy took this in stride to help keep food on the table and the many mouths fed.

Guiding Questions:

- What resonated with you?

- Butch was creative with an inquisitive mind. In what ways are you curious, creative, and inquisitive?

- How do you use your curiosity and creativity in your life?

- What question do you need to ask yourself but are afraid of the answer?

- Butch always had a smile on his face and ready hands to help his family. How do you greet your family when they ask you for help?

- Butch Cassidy worked on ranches close to home to help support his family. What are two new things you could do to support your family?

- How does it enrich your life when you help someone?

- Money has a story of its own that runs in the background of our decision making. These stories are so quiet that we don't even realize that we're making decisions related to money most of the time. What stories do you hear running in the background of Butch's story?

- How did these shadow stories drive his decisions?

- How did money stories affect the family's decision making?

- What shadow stories affect your decisions around money?

- What financial decisions do you need to pay more attention to?

- There are many things influencing our spending habits. We see basic survival needs in Leroy's story like feeding his family. We also see a desire for adventure. What other shadow stories do you hear in his story?

CHAPTER 5
HARDSHIP & COMMUNITY

Robert Leroy Parker's parents, Anne and Maximillian, were part of The Great Mormon Migration, who answered Brigham Young's call to come to America to settle the great state of Utah. As immigrants from England, they had to cross over a thousand miles of wilderness including the area now know as Wyoming. The drive West came quickly and unexpectedly for many Mormons. They had only just recently settled in the Missouri area when the governor at the time issued an executive order that allowed the execution of Mormons. This lead to the move out West quickly without time to prepare.

They, most likely, were among 70,000 immigrants who followed the Sweetwater River from Independence Rock to South Pass. Crossing the Continental Divide through the Rocky Mountains, they crossed the beautiful state of Wyoming. Here they found plenty of water and good pasture for their livestock. The gentle slope out of South Pass made the valley a good choice through the mountains. They dubbed it "crossing the elephant's spine."

Thousands of immigrants crossed Wyoming. Some made it, some didn't. Covered wagons were a luxury that many could not afford. Don't let your imagination fool you. The long wagon convoys often seen in Hollywood films were rare for many of the poor immigrants heading West to try and stake their claim. For most this journey was undertaken on foot, brutal and grueling. A young Brigham Young envisioned human-powered handcarts as the key to moving West. This idea proved to be one of the most brilliant – and tragic – experiments in all Western emigration.

Regardless, thats what they were outfitted with, handcarts. To bring this image into your imagination, these human-powered wagons were nothing more than just a fancy way of saying a wooden wheelbarrow. The standard handcart box measured three feet by four feet, with eight inch walls centered over a single axle with a wagon-style wheels on both sides. Between two stabilizing handles, extending out front was a cross bar for one adult to push on with all their might. The pushed into the cross bar pulling the handcart along the trail.

Fully loaded, the handcart could hold around 500 pounds of provisions and possessions. Each individual adult was allowed 17 pounds of clothing and bedding. Children were allowed 10 pounds. When things got onerous along the trail, belongings were quickly pitched along the road, each new obstacle called into reality a battle of values. This was all they owned. Was the item important to life, was the value provided worth the pain and challenge to drag its weight? Keep in mind all of this was pulled by one adult, with possibly a couple of kids hitching a ride.[1] To make this already challenging mode of transportation all the more intense due to the extermination order issued in Missouri, the carts at the time were mostly made out of green wood. Green wood is problematic because as it ages and the water evaporates out, cracks and splinters in unexpected and potentially disastrous ways.

There is no doubt that the 1300 mile journey was hard on the travelers and their beasts of burden, if they had any at all. The routes were chosen for the ease of livestock, not the people. Weather could make all the difference in their success or failure. If the caravan left too early in the

---

[1] https://history.churchofjesuschrist.org/content/trek/iowa-city-1856?lang=eng

spring, that meant less food for the livestock. If they departed too late, then many became trapped in the mountains by heavy snowfall.[2]

The brave souls marched by day facing great danger and overcoming hardships. But at night, the pioneers told stories and danced[3] by the light of their campfires. This was a time to celebrate that they were alive. Living through such trying circumstances built a lot of community and camaraderie. They would need each other to survive the harsh Western frontier once they reach Utah.

Guiding Questions:

- What did you hear in the story?

- Anne and Maximillian answered a call to adventure when they left England. What call to adventure did you answer in your past?

---

[2] https://history.churchofjesuschrist.org/content/historic-sites/wyoming/remembering-handcart-pioneers-in-the-sweetwater-valley?lang=eng

[3] https://scholarsarchive.byu.edu/cgi/viewcontent.cgi?article=2144&context=inscape#:~:text=Dance is not found in,of dance in contemporary Mormondom.

- Ann and Macmillan had to manage many hardships, including harsh conditions, difficult choices, and letting go of things they value, as well as the possibility of death. What hardships do you have to navigate if you accept the call to your adventure?

- What do you need to do to begin the adventure?

- How has accepting a call to adventure lead you to a purpose?

- What purpose is giving your life meaning now?

- What call to adventure have you been ignoring that you need to pay attention to?

- The Great Mormon Migration came with incredible hardship. Brigham Young successfully migrated thousands of Mormons to Utah. How do you think the hardship along the way helped prepare them to settle Utah?

- How has hardship in the past prepared you for challenges you face now in your life?

- Being a part of The Great Mormon Migration, you can imagine the importance they must have given to this purpose, fleeing the execution orders. This purpose, and their religious values, gave them the grit and determination to keep going and achieve their goal. How do your values relate to significant experiences in your life?

- How does purpose help you carry on through the hard times to achieve your goals?

- What purpose or values can you tap into to help you achieve your true north?

- The travelers pitched items when their load became to heavy. What do you need to "pitch" from your life to make your life easer?

- Untranslatable words resonate with us because we recognize them in our own lives. The Japanese untranslatable word, *kanso* means living with and acting upon the simplicity and clarity that may be achieved through the elimination of clutter. It is the willingness to remove the non-essential elements that get in the way of your success as well as the willingness to part with the things that do not serve you. How would eliminating the clutter make your life better?

- The travelers worked hard during the day, facing great danger, but they found time to tell stories and dance by the campfire. The harsh realities faced day-to-day brought a sense of relief. Given the survival of their community, their relief gave way to a celebration each evening. How do you take time to find joy, even when times are hard, in a way that strengthens your bonds to family, friends, or community?

- How does navigating hardships with a community behind you relate to your challenge, essential question, and big idea?

- What additional guiding resources do you need to navigate hardships?

- How do the hardships relate to your true north?

CHAPTER 6
A BAD TASTE

The law was rough and tumble on the Western frontier. Sheriffs were few and law enforcement often relied on the local population to support them when they had to apprehend outlaws. Some citizens weren't fans of the local law and supported the outlaws. No matter what side of the law you were on, it was a dangerous life. The line between the two was often thinly veiled. It didn't take long for Leroy to get into trouble. His first offense was minor, but it is said that it left him resentful towards the legal system and people in authority.

One day, after a long dusty ride into town, Leroy arrived at the local store to buy a pair of pants. When he found the store closed, he was irritated and mighty disappointed. So, without further ado, he decided to let himself in and take a look around. He helped himself to a piece of pie and found the pair of pants he was looking for. After he was finished eating his pie and shopping for his pants, he left an IOU. He was planning to return with the payment next time he was in town. With his to do list successfully completed he went on his merry way back home.

Well, when the store owner opened the next day, they were not pleased to find an IOU. The store owner wasn't having any of that! He marched right over the sheriff's office and pressed charges against that boy. The sheriff set out to arrest young Leroy for theft. Although he was let go, Leroy wasn't going to forget how he was treated, he was 13 years old at the time of his first arrest. This experience set the stage for the rest of his life. He carried this memory with him, which was reflected in his attitude towards the law, for his entire life.

Guiding Questions:

* What resonated with you?

* Leroy was trying to find a creative solution to his need. He had a loose understanding of commerce practices. He thought he had found a workable solution. How did making assumptions without checking to see if they are true affect his decision making?

- How might acting on an assumption without checking to see if it was true affecting your decision making?

- Creative problem solving stems from the ability to approach problems in novel ways and develop innovative solutions that go beyond conventional thinking. Butch's creative problem solving was certainly in full process. He was thinking out-of-the-box, but he didn't seek feedback on his idea. How do you use creativity to try and find alternative solutions to obstacles?

- What challenge are your facing that you need to use creative problem solving currently?

- Whose feedback do you need on your creative problem solving?

- In 1984, researcher Laurence Kohlberg posed the following story. We often see a version of this story in movies, books, and we experience them in real life. As you read this short story make notes of your observations. There are no right or wrong answers.

  A man's wife is dying of cancer and there is only one drug that can save her. The only place to get the drug is at the store of a pharmacist who is known to overcharge people for drugs. The man can only pay $1,000, but the pharmacist wants $2,000, and refuses to sell it to him for less, or to let him pay later. Desperate, the man later breaks into the pharmacy and steals the medicine. How would you gauge the actions taken by the individual in this story?

- What do you notice about your response to the story?

- Leroy carried certain memories which shaped his attitude for the rest of his life. What shapes your outlook on life?

- How do you think Butch's story would change if the shop owner hadn't pressed charges?

- How might your life change if you made an adjustment to one attitude you have?

- There was a complete lack of communication between Leroy and the store owner. Leroy felt like he had communicated clearly that he would be back with payment. The store owner did not find this satisfactory. How do you facilitate conversation with those around you?

- What conversations do you need to have to attain retain the support you need to remain on course with your true north?

- Whose feedback might be helpful as you explore your essential question?

CHAPTER 7
BECOMING BUTCH CASSIDY

Life on the range was tough and employment could be volatile. The cattle industry was big money run by powerful cattle barons in the late 1800's. Smaller ranches had to be tough to survive. One of those was the Marshal Ranch not far from Leroy's home in Utah. Here he met his boyhood hero Mike Cassidy. Mike took Leroy under his wing and taught him all about cowboying. He looked after the younger Leroy teaching him all about horses and guns. These skills would prove to be vital for the rest of his life.

Mike Cassidy was a small time rustler. It was easy for cowboys to fall into rustling after a lean year. Before long, he got caught. Off he went to prison, his path never crossed with the young Leroy again. Between Leroy's brush with law and Mike Cassidy getting hauled off, that was enough for Leroy to think about his future differently. The boy used his imagination to visualize a different life.

Leroy loved his family and highly valued the importance of family. In 1884 the local law came looking for some cattle rustlers. Being a young man who knew the locals well, he had an inkling of who the rustlers were that the law was looking for. Knowing that they were family men trying to take care of their families, Leroy took the blame for the crime and fled town. He knew that his life would be limited, only scrapping by. But Leroy always saw the bright side of a problem. He saw an opportunity to leave the limits of his poor existence behind. He took the blame setting Leroy on a path of crime. He left his family and the community he grew up with but it is said that he carried them with him as well a valuable lessons and skills.

Leroy did not take long to up his game. In 1889 Leroy, along with two other men were suspected of robbing the Telluride Bank. This daring raid took him into the spotlight with a new level of crime. This recent development with the law got him to thinking. He needed to protect his family and the best way to do that is to change his name. In honor of his boyhood hero and the first outlaw he knew, Leroy took Cassidy as his last name. He assumed the name George to further separate himself from his family.

Leroy struck out on his own, flush with cash. For a while he tried to stay true to the law. He worked as a butcher in Rock Springs, Wyoming, quickly becoming a steady and neighborly addition to the community. His friendly way with people caught the attention of his neighbors and they started calling him Butch.[4] The name stuck and he became known as Butch Cassidy.

Guiding Questions:

- What resonated with you?

---

[4] https://www.history.com/news/6-things-you-might-not-know-about-butch-cassidy

- Mike Cassidy had a significant impact on young Leroy. How do you decide to allow someone to influence you?

- Butch's early experiences on ranches and his brushes with the law shaped his decisions toward becoming an outlaw. How has your experiences shaped you?

- Butch's turn towards a career of crime forced him to leave his family behind. What have you left behind?

- Butch changed his name to protect his family. Who do you need to protect and what do you need to do to protect them?

- Butch left his mother's religion behind but carried many of her values and what he had learned from her. What do you carry with you?

- How do you see Butch evolving?

- How do you see yourself evolving?

- What turn do you need to take to stay on course towards your true north?

- Butch turned towards a life of crime. How do you know this is the right turn to take towards your true north?

CHAPTER 8
BEEF BUBBLE

Butch, as he was now known, was restless and wanted to build a better life for himself. Wyoming was in the heyday of the "beef bubble." Those early days were something else. The papers called the profits astonishing, especially in the Wyoming Territory.

In those days the Wyoming grass was abundant and exceedingly nutritious, ideal for large herds of cattle. On account of the heavy snow and wet winters, good water was everywhere. When it came time to send the cows to market, the railroad provided cheap transportation east to market. Just over the yonder pass, all around Cheyenne and up through the heart of Wyoming, in 1885 you could find an 1.5 million cattle grazing.

Now this beef bubble, had huge profits, attracting the attention of many powerful people That included territorial governors, the military, businessmen, cattlemen who invested in livestock, along with the many confidants and those looking for the highlife. The cattlemen soon become cattle barons who created the Wyoming Stock Growers Association, the most powerful political organization in the West.

Cattlemen fanned out all across the Wyoming Territory, staking out ranches across the vast plains of Wyoming with millions of dollars of cattle kept pouring in.[5] For a young man seeking a better life, the money flowing in and out of Wyoming and the surrounding areas, was pretty tempting.

---

[5] https://www.wyohistory.org/encyclopedia/wyoming-cattle-boom-1868-1886#:~:text=On May 1, 1867, Cheyenne,Good water was "everywhere."

Guiding Questions:

- What resonated with you?

- Wyoming has always been a boom-bust state with its reliance on natural resources. During the beef bubble, the wet winters brought an abundance of grass and water needed for raising cattle and easy access to cheap transportation with the railroads. Today it is the reliance on energy resources. What natural resources do you have that might be causing a boom-bust cycle in your life?

- Booms typically follow years of bust. What hardships have you endured before you had your boom?

- How did the bust prepare you for the boom?

- According to research published in the Journal of the Association of Consumer research, a scarcity mindset is a deep seeded belief that your resources are limited and there is not enough to go around. This focuses your attention on mitigating risk and hoarding resources. The abundance mindset is founded on a belief that there are enough resources to go around with abundant opportunities for collaboration and innovation. This leads to confidence, creativity and collaboration. This abundant mindset tends to focus your attention on taking chances and pursuing opportunities to grow. How might a scarcity or abundant mindset work for you?

- In Sweden, the word *Lagom* describes the self-awareness of being able to differentiate between what is essential in your life and when something is no longer serving you. Knowing this difference can help you to embrace what is good enough. Instead of buying things to fulfill you, *Lagom* suggests that finding pleasure and fulfillment comes with moderation. It is about making choices that require a bit of personal sacrifice to benefit the world. For you, how does this Swedish word relate to a scarcity or abundant mindset?

- If we look at money as not actually a thing but an unconscious agreement between us that lives within a society, what have you unconsciously agreed to in your mind when you spend money?

- Money is fickle. How do you avoid living your life to acquire things you don't need?

- How do you need to use money to manifest your true north?

CHAPTER 9

THE SIDEKICK

A gawky teenager named Harry Alonzo Longabaugh left his home in Pennsylvania to seek his fortune in the wild West. With visions in his head of becoming a cowboy, he high tailed it west but finding work as a ranch hand was scarce, especially for a scrawny 15 year old teenager without any experience.

In those days when you bought a horse, there wasn't the paperwork or bill of sale we are accustomed to today. You just handed over the cash and took off on the horse.

The Western territories were a tough place with the big ranchers protecting their holdings. They were not above using their own trickery and thievery to keep control, money, and power within their hands. When one of those barons wanted to make their point, they may sell a horse to a smaller rancher or a cowboy. Because it was a good ole' boys network, they headed down to the Sheriff's office and reported a theft, a crime punishable by death. They got their horse back and kept the money.

So it happened that young Harry Lonabaugh came across such a challenging situation. He was accused of horse thieving in Sundance, Wyoming. History, we don't know if he actually stole the horse or if it was nothing more than a cheap way for some big rancher to make some money and keep his property.

Horse thieving was a hanging offense, but instead of going to the gallows, Harry went to jail for two years. It was in jail that he is rumored to have picked up his nickname. Some people say it was because he was so young when he was arrested, others say it was because he committed the crime in Sundance. This encounter with the law earned Harry a nickname that he would carry with him for the rest of his notorious career. Young Harry Lonabaugh became known as the Sundance Kid.

And don't go thinking that he was a stone cold killer like some say. After his release he became famous for his skills with a gun. However, the newspapers of the time sensationalized his exploits. Both Butch Cassidy and the Sundance Kid had an aversion to killing.6 There is no documented killings for either of them, or the Wild Bunch Gang for that mater. In reality, the Sundance Kid only served time for stealing a horse when he was scrawny teenager, years before he earned his notoriety.

But we're getting ahead of ourselves. Butch Cassidy and the Sundance Kid didn't meet until several years after they both had been released from jail.

Guiding Questions:

• What did you hear in this part of the story?

---

6 https://www.oldwest.org/the-sundance-kid/

- The legacy of Butch Cassidy and the Sundance Kid have linked these two men together for over 160 years. With whom are you linked?

- If you were to write your obituary that would be read for 160 years, what do you want your legacy to highlight?

- The wild west was known to be lawless. The rich ranchers of the time were as lawless as the outlaws. How do you think they were similar?

- How do you think the ranchers and outlaws are different?

- The media of the time sensationalized the exploits of Butch and Sundance, clouding the truth even to today. How do you know what is real and what is sensationalized in the news today?

- How do you protect yourself from fake news?

- How do you evaluate who is whispering in your ear?

- Who do you need by your side while you explore your essential question and make progress towards your challenge?

CHAPTER 10
PINKERTON DETECTIVE AGENCY

Butch Cassidy loved Wyoming! Depending on who you listen to, some say Butch and Wyoming didn't get along too well. I bet that rumor was spread by none other than the Pinkerton Detective Agency.

The Pinkerton Detective Agency was established in the 1850s by Allan Pinkerton, an immigrant from Glasgow, Scotland who grew up poor with a fire in his belly. Towards the end of his life, he wrote a popular book series based on his agency's most famous cases. He explained his accomplishments by citing "well-directed and untiring energy" and "a determination not to yield until success was assured."7

For six years Butch eluded the most powerful detectives on the planet. E.H. Harriman, owner of the Union Pacific Railroad, hired the Pinkerton Detective Agency to track down Butch, Sundance, and the Wild Bunch Gang after they had pulled off a string of rapid-fire robberies. They hit trains and banks before disappearing overnight into the wilderness. The local sheriff's were continually coming up empty handed. The local communities were ambivalent about helping the law catch the Wild Bunch Gang. Between Butch's charisma and his generous helping hand secured an unprecedented network of friends willing to throw law enforcement off their trail.

The railroad companies were not going to let Butch and the Wild Bunch Gang get away with stealing from them. They hired private muscle to defend them from their thievery. Now these fellas were good, and I mean really good! They were known worldwide for their toughness as well as their ruthless, effective, and novel investigative tactics. When the Federal

---

7 https://www.smithsonianmag.com/history/outlaw-hunters-163405565/

Bureau of Investigation (FBI) was founded, they based their model on the Pinkerton Detective Agency.

With such a star studded reputation for capturing outlaws, why couldn't they catch Butch? That is a good question. These guys were motivated to claim the legendary Butch and Sundance for the bragging rights. One of their agents was quoted saying that they thought that Cassidy was the most skilled and daring outlaw of the time. A time when many other notorious outlaws ran rampant across the West like Jesse James, Billy the Kid, Belle Starr, and the Texan gunfighter John Wesley Hardin.

So when Butch and Sundance slipped through their fingers and rumors began to spread that they were in South America, I'm guessing The Pinkerton Detective Agency was pretty motivated to let everyone believe that they were killed in Bolivia.

Butch was known as a criminal mastermind. If he was so smart pulling off those robberies and elusive enough to evade the best detective agency in the world, does it make sense that they were captured in South America?8 Or was it another genius plot to create a diversion so Butch and Sundance could slip out of the limelight and elude the law once more?

So who do you think told all those stories about Butch and Sundance being shot up in South America? Well the Pinkerton Detective Agency certainly wouldn't be motivated to say anything different. They would have pie all over their faces.

---

8 https://www.history.com/news/6-things-you-might-not-know-about-butch-cassidy

Guiding Questions:

- What resonated with you?

- Who do you think told all those stories about Butch and Sundance being shot up in South America?

- The papers reported that Butch and Sundance were killed in South America. Here in Wyoming, many report that Butch came back here to visit after those articles. His own family reports that he didn't die in South America. What do you believe?

- How do you validate your own assumptions?

- In the last few years, what was believed to be the bodies of Butch and Sundance in Bolivia were exhumed and given DNA tests. It was found that they were not a DNA match to them. How does this information change your perspective?

- Figuring out what is a credible source of information was difficult back then. It is still true today. Misinformation can be devastating to your health, wellness, and well-being. How do you decide what sources are credible?

- How has gossip influenced Butch and Sundance's story?

- How do you handle gossip?

- Butch was one of the most successful outlaws of the wild west. He is thought to be a criminal mastermind. As the brains behind the success of their robberies, Butch would meticulously study their goal and plan out the robbery down to the weight of the bounty (ie:silver, gold) and how it would affect the horses during their escape. What are your thoughts about this kind of detailed planning?

- How would you take these insights and apply it to your own goal setting and planning?

- Allan Pinkerton, the founder of the Pinkerton Detective Agency still in business today, wrote something similar about his own success. He believed in showing respect to his adversity. In his pursuit of his goal, he attributes his success to "well-directed and untiring energy" and "a determination not to yield until success was assured." How do you decide when it is time to quit?

- Thomas Edison said, "The trouble with most people is that they quit before they start." What do you need to start?

- Thomas Jefferson pointed out, "If you want something you have never had, you must be willing to do something you have never done." What is "it" that waits for you and what do you need to "do?"

- Research shows that if you have a written plan, you will manage setbacks and disappointments better. What is your plan for setbacks and disappointments?

- How would a written plan affect your challenge, essential question and big idea?

CHAPTER 11
SPIRITUALITY & TRUST

Mrs. Slosson arranged for Miss Mary Gates to conduct music during the services. They brought in the best local talents they could find. The prisoners seemed anxious to go to these services instead of making up excuses as they did before they came to the prison. These two remarkable women made their mark on the hearts and minds of the inmates. Another woman of note who assisted within the Wyoming Territorial Prison was Miss Fannie Marsh. She is believed to be the first woman to work along side convicts in any penitentiary system. She was a pianist who would come in on occasion and play music for the inmates.

Guiding Questions:

- What resonated with you?

- Mrs. Slosson and Miss Gates had a passion for spirituality, music, and education. Following that passion, they made the difference in a lot of people's lives. How do you allow your passion to fuel your drive?

- Mrs. Slosson and Miss Gates pioneered women working with prisoners. They were unafraid of pursuing what they wanted. They walked boldly into the unknown. How do you engage with the unknown?

- Mrs. Slosson and Miss Gates became leaders without the title. What opportunities do you have to show leadership?

- Peter Nulty, wrote in Fortune Magazine, "Of all the skills of leadership, listening is the most valuable – and one of the least understood. Most captains of industry listen only sometimes, and they remain ordinary leaders. But a few, the great ones, never stop listening. That's how they get word before anyone else of unseen problems and opportunities." What do you believe Mrs. Slosson and Miss Gates heard when they listened beyond the superficial?

- Cheryl, Richardson wrote, "People start to heal the moment they feel heard." When you feel heard, how does that change your behavior?

- Deborah Tannen of Georgetown University wrote, "To say that a person feels listened to means a lot more than just their ideas get heard. It's a sign of respect. It makes people feel valued." Whose life could you change by listening?

- To put a finer point on it, an unknown author said, "You don't have to save me, you just have to hold my hand while I save myself." How would your world change if you dedicated time to hold someone's hand and listen to them?

- Mrs. Slosson and Miss Gates wanted to bring services that would improve the lives of the inmates. They saw people in need, they heard their pain, and believed they could help using their own unique knowledge and skills. What unique knowledge and skills do you have that you are willing to bring to serving others?

- Science reveals that volunteering is good for your health. Those who volunteer have a lower mortality rate than those who do not. Older volunteers tend to walk more, find it easier to cope with everyday tasks, and less likely to develop high blood pressure, and they have better thinking skills. Audrey Hepburn said, "As you grow older, you will discover that you have two hands – one for helping yourself, the other for helping others." In other words, if you fill one hand with volunteering, then you fill the other one with helping yourself. What are you doing with your hands?

- Desmond Tutu observed, "Do your little bit of good where you are; it's those little bits of good that put together overwhelm the world." What little bits of good are you putting into the world?

- Mrs. Slosson brought community to the prison. Community is also critical to healing from trauma. Where do you find community?

- Mahatma Gandhi said, "The best way to find yourself is to lose yourself in the service of others." What does service mean to you?

- How could you expand your mind by being in service to others?

- "There can be no greater gift than that of giving one's time and energy to helping others without expecting anything in return." - Nelson Mandela. How do you give your time and energy to others without expecting anything in return?

- How does focusing on others relate to your big idea?

- How does focusing on others further your challenge?

- In their time, Mrs. Slosson and Miss Gates were not given the right to work in prisons. They changed the prison system of their time and the experience of the inmates. How are being in service to to others, listening, and a good community related?

CHAPTER 12
BALL AND CHAIN

Perhaps it was the early influence of his mentor Mike Cassidy, or maybe he just gave into temptation with all that money flowing through the Wyoming territory. What brought Butch to the Laramie State Penitentiary was a $5 grand larceny charge for stealing a horse. He had not yet become the leader of the Wild Bunch Gang or met up with the Sundance Kid. He simply bought a horse that had been stolen. This information was suppressed during his trial.

When Butch arrived at the penitentiary he wasn't shackled like the other prisoners. Warden Adams wanted to know why Butch had such a liberty. The story goes that the night before he went to jail, that smooth talking Butch convinced the Court Clerk to let him out so he could take care of some unfinished business. He promised to be back by daylight. The Clerk told the jail deputy, "If Cassidy said so, he'll keep his word." Well low and behold, there was Butch at dawn ready to do his time. Sheriff Charlie Stough seemed to have a similar trust in Butch, he escorted him to Laramie along with five other prisoners but Butch was the only one who was not secured by a ball and chain. When the warden asked Butch why he came back, he remarked, "there's honor among thieves."

The ball and chain, attached to a prisoner's leg, was one type of punishment implemented in the prison. A 20 pound ball on a short chain made it mighty difficult to walk. You couldn't just stroll along dragging that ball around. You had to carry it.

Guiding Questions:

• What resonated with you?

• The ball and chain was a type of punishment implemented in prison. What ball and chain are your carrying?

- How does that ball and chain imprison you?

- People trusted Butch because he had empathy for other people. He did what he said he was going to do. Because of his reputation, he did not have to wear the ball and chain. What actions do you need to take to release yourself from the ball and chain?

- Butch may have been a criminal but he was considered honorable. How do you reconcile these two thoughts?

- The clerk and the sheriff are two examples of people who made exceptions for Butch because they believed him to be honorable. How do you change your actions when you believe someone to be honorable?

- How do you act honorably with those around you?

- To this day, people believe Butch to be honorable. What does it mean to you to keep your word?

- What do you believe to be the impact of reputation?

- What changes do you need to make on your path towards your true north?

CHAPTER 13
FORGIVENESS

January 20, 1896, Governor William Richards pardoned the convicted rustler Butch Cassidy after he had served a year and half of his two year sentence. Judge Knight sent a letter to Governor Richards requesting a pardon in good faith. He called Butch a brave, daring fellow and a man well calculated to be a leader, and should his inclinations run that way, he would be capable of organizing and leading a lot of desperate men to desperate deeds.

It is rumored that Butch learned of the guilty verdict before the jury returned or the verdict was made public. A friend offered him horses and a means to escape but at the time he said he believed Judge Knight as an honest man and would not be governed by the wishes of those whom he believed were persecuting him instead of prosecuting him. He decided to stay and take his sentence.

Butch wrote the judge a note saying that he had no cause to complain and that he had received justice, thanking him for giving him a fair trail.[9]

Butch's friendly character was legendary, his reputation carrying him far even in the early days. In addition to knowing Judge Knight, he was friends with the prosecuting attorney Will Simpson. The petition sent to the governor was written from the citizens of Fremont County, the county that Butch had been arrested. The Governor of Wyoming famously gave Butch a pardon with the agreement that he would keep his criminal activity away from the great state of Wyoming.

---

[9] https://wyostatearchives.wordpress.com/2016/01/19/on-this-day-in-wyoming-history-butch-cassidy-is-pardoned-1896/#:~:text=Wyomin

Guiding Questions:

- What resonated with you?

- Judge Knight, Govrenor William Richards, friends who offered him a means of escape, the prosecuting attorney Will Simpson, and the citizens of Fremont County all advocated for Butch. Who has advocated for you in the past or present, and how did you respond to that kindness?

- "The greatest prison people live in is the fear of what other people think." David Icke. What do you hear in this quote?

- How does fear affect your life?

- How can you let the shackles of fear fall away?

- "I have walked that long road to freedom. I have tried not to falter; I have made missteps along the way. But I have discovered the secret that after climbing a great hill, one only finds that there are many more hills to climb. I have taken a moment here to rest, to look back on the distance I have come. But I can only rest for a moment, for with freedom comes responsibilities, and I dare not linger for my long walk is not ended." - Nelson Mandela. Life is a journey that has many hills along the way. How do you appreciate where you have come from and allow that to carry you further?

- In the quote, Nelson Mandela described taking a moment to rest and look back on the distance he has come. A time, with a relaxed mind, he can reflect on the lessons learned, so that he may apply those insights to his journey forward. How do you take time to reflect with a relaxed mind on lessons learned?

- With freedom comes responsibility. How do you care for the responsibility of your freedom?

- What does freedom mean to you?

Take some time to contemplate this poem and what it means to you.

The Road Not Taken by Robert Frost

Two roads diverged in a yellow wood,

And sorry I could not travel both

And be one traveler, long I stood

And looked down one as far as I could

To where it bent in the undergrowth;

Then took the other, as just as fair,

And having perhaps the better claim,

Because it was grassy and wanted wear;

Though as for that the passing there

Had worn them really about the same,

And both that morning equally lay

In leaves no step had trodden black.

Oh, I kept the first for another day!

Yet knowing how way leads on to way,

I doubted if I should ever come back.

I shall be telling this with a sigh

Somewhere ages and ages hence:

Two roads diverged in a wood, and I —

I took the one less traveled by,

And that has made all the difference.

Guiding Questions:

- What does this poem mean to you?

- When have you traveled the road less traveled?

- Joseph Campbell said, "If you can see your path laid out in front of you step by step, you know it's not your path. Your own path you make with every step you take. That's why it's your path." Whose path are you on?

- Forgiveness is a powerful word. Many people seek forgiveness. The issue with forgiveness is that one must be wronged in order to give it. What does forgiveness mean to you?

- How do you handle forgiveness?

- What are the advantages of not taking either road?

- What are the disadvantages of not taking either road?

- What are the disadvantages of each road?

- What are the advantages of each road?

- What path do you need to take towards your true north?

CHAPTER 14

LEADERSHIP

It's hard to tell how the time at the Wyoming Territorial Prison impacted Butch. What we do know is that he went on to be the notorious leader of the Wild Bunch Gang. Several other inmates who served alongside Butch would later become suspected members or supporters of the Wild Bunch Gang.

It was Butch's meticulous planning that made his robberies so successful. According to an article printed in the magazine Wild West, "Little was left to chance. Butch and a few selected gang members would spend days, sometimes weeks, scouting a robbery site and the best escape route. Wisely, they always chose the summer months for all their holdups, when the weather was favorable for eluding posses.

It appears that Butch also avoided killing. Although shots were fired during escapes, he was never known to have shot anyone during a holdup. The closest Butch ever came to harming a robbery victim was when he used explosives to force his way into an express car. A few express messengers were injured in the blasts, but not seriously. The gang always warned them when they would use dynamite, and the train employees were wise enough to protect themselves by hiding behind the cargo."[10]

---

[10] https://www.biography.com/crime/butch-cassidy-sundance-kid-real-story

Guiding Questions:

- What resonated with you?

- "The most dangerous people are the ignorant." – Henry Ward Beecher. How do you stay informed?

- How do you verify that you are gathering information from reputable sources?

- "In this world there is always danger for those who are afraid of it." – George Bernard Shaw. What danger do you fear that may not be the threat you think it is?

- How do you mitigate danger in your life to pursue what is important?

- "The greatest glory in living lies not in never falling, but in rising every time we fall." -Nelson Mandela: What gives you strength to rise when you fall?

- Confucius says, "He who learns but does not think, is lost. He who thinks but does not learn is in greater danger." What do you need to learn but avoid thinking about it?

CHAPTER 15

FULFILLMENT

Butch's story has come to an end; however, your story is still being written. Throughout this journal we have explored a multitude of ideas relating to your true north. Reading about the trails and tribulations that Butch faced may have stimulated new ways of looking at your life and the challenges you face. Use the guiding questions in this chapter to reflect on your journaling and formulate a framework to put into action what you have learned about yourself and your challenge so that you may reach for your north star.

- What are you learning about yourself?

- How can you apply this insight into yourself to your true north?

- "It is what we make out of what we have been given, not what we are given, that separates one person from another." - Nelson Mandela. How do you appreciate the gifts you have that separate you from others?

- "As I walked out the door toward the gate that would lead to my freedom, I knew if I didn't leave my bitterness and hatred behind, I'd still be in prison." - Nelson Mandela. What do you need to leave behind so that you can move forward?

- How do you let go of strong emotions so that they do not control your life?

- "For you to be free is not merely to cast off one's chains, but to live in a way that respects and enhances the freedom of others." - Nelson Mandela. What chains do you need to cast off to be free in mind and body?

- What choices do you need to realize your true north?What are you willing to do in the next week towards making your true north a reality?

- What barriers will you need to manage?

- Who do you need ask for support?

- What resources do you need?

- How will you celebrate your success?

Congratulations on your journey with Butch Cassidy. You have walked in his shoes, learned from his experiences and now it I sup to you to apply the insights so that you can live your best life!

ABOUT THE AUTHORS

Ryan Elledge, MA, PCC, NBHWC

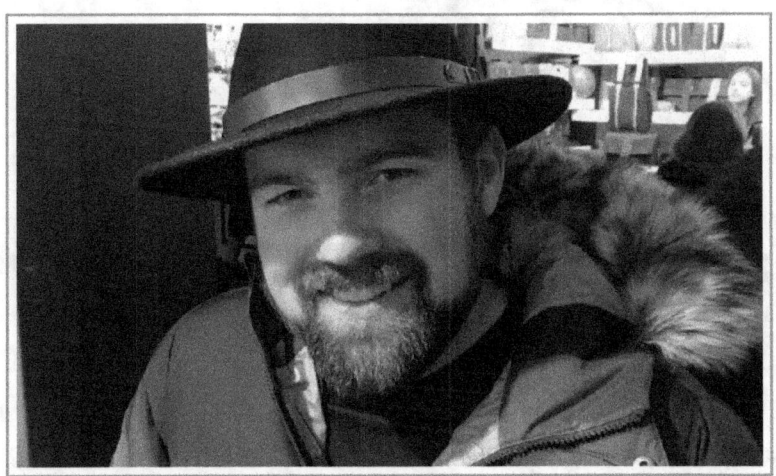

Ryan serves as a senior project manager and trainer for Mentor Agility. Concurrently, his passion for trauma-informed coaching has led him to pursue a masters in Jungian Studies, aiming to deepen his comprehensive understanding of the relationship between human psychology, trauma, and spirituality. Through his research, Ryan seeks to explore the impact of trauma-informed coaching on veterans, providing them with comprehensive support and guidance.

Ryan is a credentialed coach by the International Coaching Federation (PCC) and the National Board of Health and Wellness Coaches (NBC-HWC). He adds to his accomplishments with a personal interest in wellness as a Certified Wellness Chef and Certified Nutrition Consultant. With an undergraduate degree in agroecology, Ryan has a deep understanding of farm to table and the impact of food on wellness.

Julie Elledge, PhD, LMFT, MCC, NBHWC

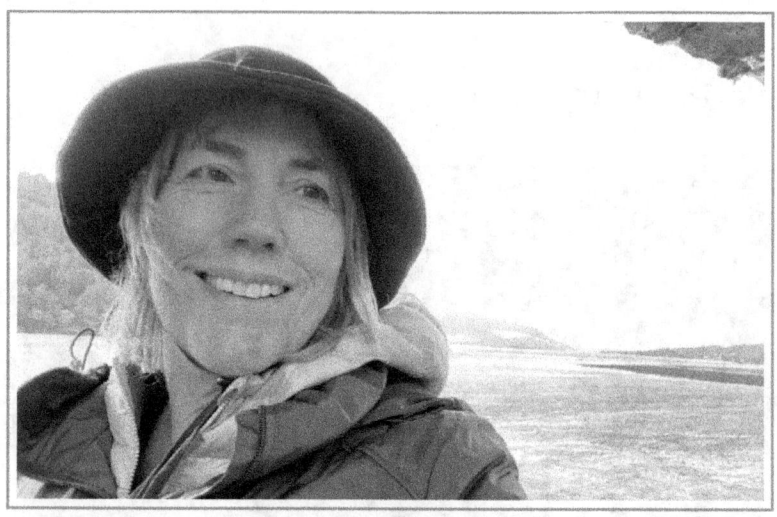

Dr. Julie Elledge has three board certifications in professional coaching: MCC , NBC-HWC, BCC. She is also a licensed family therapist, an educator with her PhD in Education, author and a recognized expert in creativity and organizational dynamics. She is the founder of Mentor Agility's Trauma-Informed Coaching Certification and the Veterans Talking to Veterans program.

She has coached in multiple disciplines for over 25 years and been an expert commentator on CyberHood Watch Radio and Fox News, among others. She has worked on education initiatives with Apple Education, Twentieth Century Fox, NOAA, BP and INEEL. Dr. Elledge offers coaching, workshops, lectures and an interdisciplinary course in NFP Leadership using the Hero's Journey® as a guide.